The Great Depression, WWII, and a Medical Miracle

In the Life of Dave Dumond

By
David D. Dumond

INFINITY
PUBLISHING

ISBN 978-0-7414-6542-9 Paperback
ISBN 978-0-7414-9402-3 eBook

Printed in the United States of America

Published September 2012

INFINITY PUBLISHING
1094 New DeHaven Street, Suite 100
West Conshohocken, PA 19428-2713
Toll-free (877) BUY BOOK
Local Phone (610) 941-9999
Fax (610) 941-9959
Info@buybooksontheweb.com
www.buybooksontheweb.com

Table of Contents

Chapter 1

My Preschool Years Growing Up on the Farm........ 1

Chapter 2

Elementary School and World War II..................... 9

Chapter 3

My High School Years... 14

Chapter 4

The After Graduation Years.................................. 18

Chapter 5

The Decision Making Years 25

Chapter 6

Our Family Business 37

Chapter 7

Those Retirement Years 45

CHAPTER 1

My Preschool Years
Growing Up on the Farm

In 1861 my grandfather James Dumond established a homestead in Shiawassee County, New Haven Township, in the State of Michigan. This is in central Lower Michigan, between Flint and Lansing the capital of Michigan. He married my grandmother Nora Hawn and together they had five children.

My father Hugh Hawn Dumond was born in 1898. In 1923 Father married my mother Marjorie Ailene Swarthout. My grandparents lived in 2 rooms in the front of the house, and my parent lived in the back and upstairs. My grandfather James passed away in 1930. Grandmother continued to live in the front two rooms of the house. My father continued to work the farm for my grandmother. I was born three days after Christmas on December 28, 1931.

The farm consisted of 70 acres of workable land. We raised milking cows, chickens, pigs, and had two workhorses for pulling the farm machinery. We would raise a steer each year for meat. My father would take bags of wheat to a waterwheel powered mill on the river in Corunna to have the wheat ground into flour. Mother would bake four or five loaves of bread every week. I had many a meal of bread and milk, and especially liked the bread with apple butter. Butter was rationed during the war. Mother would make jelly when the berries and grapes were in seasons. My grandmother could make good apple jelly.

Every Friday evening we would go into Owosso to shop and buy groceries. The big thing was sitting in the car and watching the people walking by.

In the spring my dog, Lucky a collie, and I would go to the woods on a neighbor's farm and play. I picked flowers for my mother and grandmother. My grandmother in the spring would have me bring her puffball mushrooms to cook.

I kept a drinking cup in the cow stable. When dad was milking the cows I could have warm milk to drink.

My Grandmother and I played checkers and dominoes a lot.

In the spring we would buy 200 straight run chicks. When they grew up, the pullets were kept for eggs, and the roosters were for eating and selling. When the chicks were small, they were put in a small building called a brooder coup. There was a four foot heated cover to keep the checks warm.

We purchased a special prepared chick feed for the baby chickens to eat along with water for them to drink. As the chickens grew and started to get feathers, we took the heater out. The chickens continued to grow and grow feathers. When they got large enough we moved them into a range shelter. It was built on a couple of skids, so we could move it around in the field. It was 10ft. by 12ft. with a chicken wire floor and chicken wire sides and a metal roof.

The first few evenings we would go out and drive the chickens into the shelter and shut the door to protect the chickens from animals. One evening grandma came out to help drive the chickens in. She was carrying a dust mop. One chicken tried to go by her, she threw the mop and knocked the chicken out, it lay there for a few seconds, got up and went in with rest of the chickens.

Our nearest neighbors were over a half a mile away. My dog Lucky and I played around on the farm together Cops and robbers or cowboys and Indians, we could always find something to get into. I had a swing in a high tree. There was a large tree in the back yard and it died. It was probably four feet thru at the trunk and large above. Dad cut all of the small limbs off that he could do, and left the rest for me to play on. The wood he cut was piled up to burn in the potbellied stove in our living room, the next winter.

On Saturday nights Mother would heat a pan of water on the kerosene cooking stove and put it behind the potbellied stove for me to take a bath. There was no electricity, our lights were kerosene lamps and candles, we did not have a radio or television. We used gasoline lanterns outside to do chores. I remember one Christmas I got some socks for my present, and Santa Cause left some candy and a small toy in my stocking.

I very seldom got birthday presents on my birthday. Always on Christmas

Growing wheat and oats

In the fall before the ground froze, usually the month of September, Dad would plow and work the ground with the horses preparing it to drill winter wheat. The wheat would start to grow and get green before the ground froze.

In the spring Dad would broadcast clover or alfalfa seed on the wheat ground. After the wheat was harvested, the seed grew for hay to feed the cows and horses in the winter months.

As the wheat grew, seeds began to form in the heads of the stalks. When the wheat was finished growing it dried up and turned brown. The horses then pulled a grain binder that cut the stalks off and tied the stalks in bundles. The bundles fell onto a table on the back of the binder. Dad rode on the binder and drove the horses. He would trip a lever with his foot and dump the bundles in a certain place around the field.

After the field was all cut, he would use a three-tine pitch fork and put the bundles into shocks to dry, off the ground. A neighbor farmer that had a trashing machine that was powered by a tractor would go around the neighborhood and thrash the neighborhoods wheat. All of the farmers would come with their horses and wagons to have a thrashing bee. All of the farmer's wives would come with food and share in preparing the meal for the farmers.

A huge table of doors and planks would be set up with all the food on display.

The farmers would haul the wheat from the fields to the barn with their horses and wagons. The straw was blown thru a large pipe and out the back door of the barn. My job was to walk on the straw making a straw stack of it, usually ten to twenty feet high. The wheat grain was ran into grain bags of about 100 to 120 pounds of wheat. Some of the men would put a bag on their shoulder and carry it to a granary and dumped the wheat into bins.

Oats was planted in the spring like the wheat, after the ground had thawed and started to warm up. The planting and harvesting went just like the wheat crop.

Haying

The clover and alfalfa that was sewn on the wheat field in the spring was left to grow to the next year to feed the cows and horses.

The horses would pull a mowing machine and cut the hay. After about two days when the hay was nearly dry the horses would pull a side delivery rake and put the hay into windrows.

Next, the horses would pull a wagon with a hay loader hooked behind it. The hay loader would elevate the hay up onto the wagon to my Dad and he would keep the hay leveled and stomped down.

On the front of the wagon was a standard, about two feet wide and eight feet high with steps about two feet apart. My job was to stand on the second step from the top with my knees against the top step and drive the horses. Dad would put the hay right out over my head; it was like a cave of hay. When the wagon got loaded, Dad would unhook the loader. Then he would get me out from my cave and drive the horses and wagon of hay up to the barn. Up at the barn, mother would come out to drive the horses. My father would drive the horses and wagon into the barn, unhook the horses and bring the horses back out of the barn.

Up in the top of the barn was a track that ran the full length of the barn. There was a special car on the track with a large two inch hay rope attached to it. The rope went thru a series of pulleys on the car, over to the end of the barn and down thru pulleys to the side of the barn door. The rope would be hooked to the horses.

My father would climb up on the load of hay to set two forks into the hay. I would climb up a ladder in the barn to the hay loft. Mother drove the horses pulling the hay up in the barn, when it got up in the hay loft, Dad would pull two small ropes and drop the hay in the loft. After the dust cleared I would use a three tine fork and level the hay. When the wagon got empty, we would go and get another load.

Planting and growing corn

In the spring after all frosts was out of the ground, Dad would plow the previous years hay field, work the ground down with the team of horses and prepare the ground for planting corn.

The corn was planted in rows, so we could cultivate out the weeds and grasses, keeping the corn clean. My father was able to purchase a corn husker and our first tractor to run the corn husker with a long belt from between the tractor and the husker. We built a long corncrib on the side of a tool shed. It had air spaces between the boards so the corn could dry.

When the corn was mature, Dad would cut the stalks with a corn binder pulled by the horses. Dad would sit on a seat and ride the binder, one row at a time. The binder would cut the stalks off and tie them into bundles and drop the bundles onto a table on the back of the binder. Dad would trip the table with his foot and dropped the stalks at a specified place around the field, so that the corn could be placed in shocks to dry out off the ground after several weeks when the corn was pretty dry, we would haul the bundles to the house and run them through our corn husker, removing the ears from the stalks. The ground up stalks were blown into the barn for cow feed.

I would go with father to the neighbors and husk their corn. The corn was ground up with some oats to feed the cows.

Growing navy beans for a cash crop

After the oats was harvested in the fall, Dad would work the ground and prepare it to plant navy beans in the spring. After all frost was out of the ground in May or early June in the spring, we were ready to plant white navy beans. They were drilled four rows at a time in the field so they could be cultivated just like the corn.

In the fall the beans stopped growing and the pods turned brown. We had a two-row puller pulled by the horses. It would pull two rows at a time, slicing off the roots and sliding the two rows together.

About two or three days when the pods were dry, (hoping it would not rain in this time period) we would rake two puller rows (four bean rows together). By that time, a neighbor had a bean thrasher and would come and thrash the beans, similar to the wheat harvest. This would not require as much labor as the wheat harvest. The beans were put in bins up in the granary to sell when the market price got better.

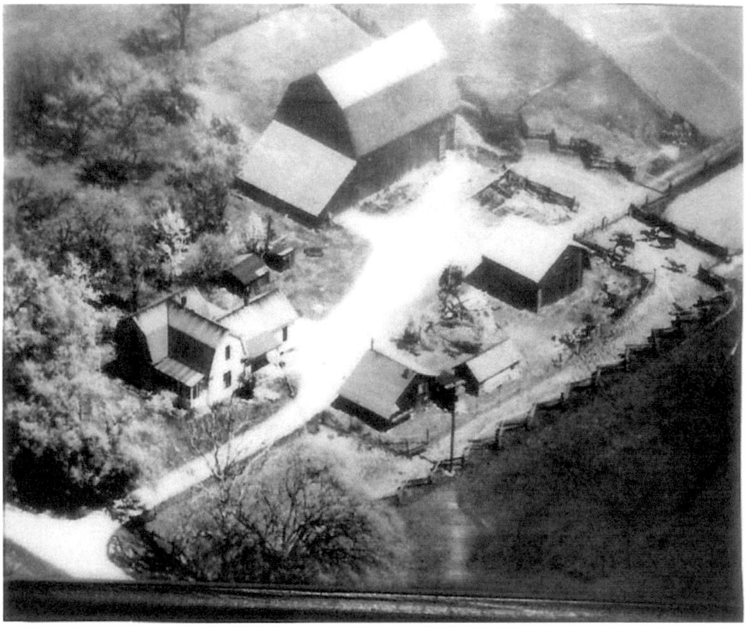

The Dumond Family Farm in the Early 1930's

CHAPTER 2

Elementary School and World War II

In the fall of 1936, at the age of five I started school. I walked one mile to school everyday. My parents took me if the weather was bad.

The school was one room with a large furnace in one corner. A woodshed in back of the school was full of wood furnished by the farmers. The teacher would start a fire in the morning, and the older boys would help keep the fire going during the day. When we came in the school, the girls would go to the right, and the boys went to the left to take off your coat, hat and boots, before entering the school. I carried a lunch bucket and a book bag for my papers and books.

There was electricity in the school. There was only one teacher for 25 to 30 students. Classes were kindergarten thru 8th grade. There was no telephone in the school. My classes during the eight years I was there were reading, writing, mathematics, health, penmanship, spelling, english, history, geography, art, citizenship, and music.

The bathrooms were two outhouses out back of the school. One for the girls and one for the boys. The students were seated by grades. There were black boards on each wall. We had a break in the morning, a break for lunch and another break in the afternoon.

On break we would go outside if the weather permitted. We would play tag, baseball, throw the ball over the school, hide and seek, racing, etc. There were swings, a slide, a merry-go-round, and teeter-totter to play on.

I remember one winter day we were sliding on the ice in the ditch out front. I fell down and hurt my shoulder. Of course there were no telephones so the teacher couldn't call my parents. The teacher tried to keep me comfortable as possible. She happened to hear the mailman stop out at the mailbox. She went out and he took me back home. I had broken my collar bone. My mother took me to the doctor.

If the weather was bad we would play games inside. After school there were kids who walked with me for the first half mile, then I turned down my road, the last half mile.

When I got home it was home work first then chores to be done. I had to feed and water the chickens (around 100) and gather the eggs. Then I would go to the barn and help my father feed the cows and horses. We would let them out every morning and evening to go up by the house and get a drink of water. There was a large iron kettle full of water for them to get a drink. We had a three inch pipe that was long enough to reach the pump by the house. My job was pumping the water for the cows and horses to drink. Then we would feed the pigs grain and water.

Next I would climb up in the hayloft, and throw down loose hay for the cows and horses. We had a small room in the barn to keep the calves in. I would get some water and mix a food supplement for them to eat. I would go out the back door of the barn and bring in straw for the cows and horses bedding.

We did not have any electricity in the buildings, we used lanterns to do the chores after dark.

Our bathroom was an outside toilet behind the house. We put the old Sears Roebuck and Montgomery catalogs out there to look at. You could look at the catalogs, then tear off a sheet to use. We had what they called a commode to use at night.

Not having any electricity we had no radio or television or video games to play. We were just coming out of the great depression and going into World War II. Gasoline was rationed for the war effort. People were issued stamps to purchase gasoline. One stamp per gallon of gas. The amount of stamps you got was based on work and essential driving, no pleasure driving.

Finally in 1941 Consumers Power Company brought electricity the ½ mile down to our farm. WOW it sure was great.

My Uncle was an electrician and helped Dad wire all of the Buildings. Prior to the electricity our water was a pump by the side of the house.

When World War II started many things happened to our country. People stepped in to help, men were drafted into the military. The women went to work in factories. Strategic items were taken to help the war effort. Butter was rationed so dad would purchase cases of apple butter to put on our bread.

All trucking became limited to strategic products only. Fruits and vegetables for instance, from the south became scarce.

You learned to substitute or do without.

Many things were done to help in the war effort. A weed called milk weed grew in fence rows and ditches throughout the farms and wetlands. In the fall they would have pods of seeds, three inches long and about one and one half inch around. Inside was a cotton like substance. This was used in the making of some things used in the military for the war effort.

Large onion sacks were delivered to rural schools. I would take some sacks and walk the fields and woods picking the pods. I would take my full sacks to school to be picked up. They gave us books to hold stickers for each sack of pods we brought in. When season was over we were given rewards for the bags of pods we turned in.

When I was in the sixth grade in the country school there was only three of us in the class, Duane, Glen and myself. In the seventh grade Glen had moved away, leaving Duane and me. For the eighth grade Duane had moved away, leaving only me. The school board decided to buss me to an elementary school in Owosso. A family that lived on the corner had me come in their house and wait for the bus each day. They were eating their breakfast at that time of morning and I could see the bus coming down the road. The class in the other school had 29 students in the 8th Grade. What an experience from the rural school

During lunch hour most of the students would go home. I carried my lunch. My teacher hired me to walk two blocks to her house and shovel her driveway and walks in the wintertime. She was nice enough to pay me each time.

Three old bachelors lived down the road. Sometimes I would go with my father on a Saturday night to watch them play cards.

One night Mother baked a cake for us to take with us. After the cake was gone one of the men set the plate on the floor for the dog to clean out. He gave me the pan and said there, you can take this home and put it in the cupboard. In a couple of days mother wanted to know if we brought the pan home. I told her yes I had put it in the cupboard. That was what they had told me to do.

CHAPTER 3

My High School Years

In 1946 I started high school at Owosso High School. I walked a half mile to the corner and rode the school bus to school. My basic course of study was vocational agriculture and business. I took bookkeeping and typing along with other required subjects. I could not participate in sports because of riding the school bus and had to do chores at home.

I got very involved with the Future Farmers of America (FFA) organization. We took many field trips to visit farms, and see different methods and procedures in farming.

We learned parliamentary procedures for public and business organizations, meeting procedures. We learned other skills such as public speaking. I would do projects at home. We would get a record book to keep track of time involved and all costs pertaining to the project. I raised a calf and kept track of the calf's daily growth, cost of feed purchased, right up to the day we started milking her as a cow.

Another project was growing popcorn for sale. I planted two acres of Austrian Hull-less popcorn. When it got ripe I would pick the corn with a corn picker, and put the corn in a crib built on posts covered with metal to prevent animals from getting at the corn. I would take about six bushel of the corn in the house, upstairs in a room with a chimney going up thru it for heat to dry the corn, after about two weeks I would shell three or four ears of the popcorn and pop it. When it would pop perfect I would take the ears of dried corn out to the barn and put the cobs through a corn sheller. I would then run the shelled popcorn over a fanning mill, complete with a screen that took out everything larger than the popcorn cornels and a screen that let every thing smaller than the cornels thru. It had a fan that blew out all light materials.

I bought plastic bags that would hold one pound of popcorn. Mother would seal the bags with her iron, after she put a card in them with my name and other information.

People all over soon found out about my popcorn and came to buy some from the guy they named the popcorn king. This was before Orville Redenbacher. Some would buy as much as ten to twenty pounds at .20 cents a pound. I sent some to other states to my customers' relatives and friends.

Of course I had to keep records of seed, fertilizer all time spent working with the popcorn and pounds sold and the profits made.

My father Hugh was very knowledgeable about many things. He could tear down an engine from a car or tractor fix it and put it back together. He was always fixing something for a neighbor. He was called the neighborhood handyman. Usually I was there helping him. We could do carpentry work and do anything that needed to be done.

As time went along we started renting more farmland from the neighbors. Some of it was for me and sometimes for dad.

We also bought newer machinery to work the farm. We bought our third tractor to work the farm. During the busy seasons Mother would help drive one of the tractors.

In my sophomore year, I had a typing class as one of my subjects. About the second week the teacher asked me to stay after class. She said all of the others teachers were wondering if I would be interested in being in charge of hall patrol, during school. It would involve going to study hall each semester and soliciting students for patrol duty at certain hall patrol desks. It was to keep students from the halls and help visitors who came to the school. She said the teachers all felt I had very good leadership abilities and would do a good job. I told her I would be glad to give it a try.

The first week I lined up students for each station, for every hour of school. After that, occasionally I would go out and check with the various hall patrol students to see if they were having any problems and if things were going OK. During my junior year the teacher called me into her class and said "they would like me to continue the hall patrol supervisors job." I said I'd be glad to. One day the teacher called me to her classroom and told me that one of the teachers had a bunch of hall patrol badges and was misusing them. She said I needed to go to him and ask for the badges. I told her I was one of his students and didn't want to. She said if he gave me a problem to come to her. He gave me all of the badges and I had no problem with him.

I continued the hall patrol supervisor's job thru my senior year also.

For all of the time spent in the agriculture projects throughout high school, I placed second in the State of Michigan Farm Mechanics Award and received a check for $25.00.

In FFA I advanced up thru several levels, from Greenhand to State Star farmer. I was recognized for the three years as hall patrol supervisor. I was presented the highest award to be presented to a graduating senior in agriculture, The Dekalb Agriculture Accomplishment Award. I got a gold medal for it.

I was also awarded an eight-week short course to Michigan State University, in the study of agriculture.

My senior year I bought a used car and drove to school. That worked out well because I was getting more involved on the farm.

I bought a used tractor for doing small jobs on the farm, cultivating, drilling, mowing, raking and pulling the wagons and doing small work around the farm. We sold the horses. The first winter I put the tractor in the heated garage and cleaned it up. I took the cultivator all apart and painted the complete tractor and tools that came with it. When I got done it looked and ran like a new tractor. I bought an arc welder for fixing machinery that broke down.

CHAPTER 4

The After Graduation Years

In 1950 my father and I formed a partnership on the farm. We had gotten rid of the horses and obtained three tractors for working the farmland. We rented an additional 180 acres from neighbors, making the total farmland to 250 acres.

We rebuilt the dairy barn, took out the plank floor and put in a concrete floor. We put in 14 new stalls for cows. We put running water for each cow. When the cows came into the barn they each had their place to go in a stall. I built a milk house with concrete blocks on the barn next to the cow stable. We purchased a machine for milking the cows. We could milk two cows at a time. We purchased a milk can cooler, it held eight milk cans that were cooled in water, and we put it in the milk house. When we finished milking a cow, we would take the milk in and put it in a can to keep it fresh. A truck came everyday and took the milk to a processing plant.

We built a special room in the barn for the small calves, when they were born. They were fed a special food we purchased and mixed with water for them. The female calves were usually kept and raised for milking cows. The male calves were sold.

We would buy two small pigs and raise them up to about 200 pounds and take them to a slaughter house to be butchered.

We had a small building to keep them in. They were fed corn and a concentrated feed we purchased for them.

I started to work with kids as a 4-H club leader. I started with a Handicraft Group. They made a lamp, and other projects of their choosing. I purchased tools and materials for them to make their projects. Their only cost was for their material.

I also had a gun safety club, working with BB guns. They were instructed in the care and handling of their guns. I was asked to take over the leadership and guidance of all 4-H clubs in New Haven Township. This would encompass girls as well as boys.

In a small town north of our farm not far from our township, they had put an outdoor swimming pool in their park. The club voted to go there as a group sometime to swim. I made arrangements for us to go there one evening. There were around 50 kids and parents there. They had a good time. I dove off the diving board and was swimming along the bottom of the pool when a boy jumped off the side and hit my neck. When I came to, three lifeguards were working over me on the side of the pool. My neck was broken. In the hospital they put a large collar around my neck. I had to wear that for several weeks.

For two years I went to a 4-H camp as a counselor for a week. We had lots of fun with the girls and boys. The kids would put on skits in the evenings. I taught them square dancing and round dancing.

I continued to have headaches and problems with my neck for a long time. I went to a chiropractor doctor for a long time.

On June 8, 1953 my grandmother passed away and the body was brought out to the farm for viewing. This was done a lot back in the earlier years, many people gathered at the farm and in the evening it got very dark outside, someone said look at the weather vane on top of the barn, the rooster was going around and around. We watched the clouds: some were coming from the northwest, another from the southwest and some from the southeast. It did not rain. The clouds moved off toward the east, they looked bad. About an hour later, my aunt and uncle came from Flint, they said a tornado had hit on Coldwater Road on the north side of Flint. This was exactly east of our farm about twenty miles.

About the middle of June 1953, a few weeks after Grandmothers Funeral, I was cultivating beans with my tractor when a thunderstorm started to come up. I went to the house and ran the tractor into the tool shed. It was raining very hard and the thunder and lightning was very sharp. I did not have a shirt on. I ran to the house between thunders, where my mother was setting on a covered porch. We talked about the storm and I said I have some things to do on my car, I'm going to put it in the garage, which was directly across the driveway from the house, and work on it.

After the next thunder, I ran to my car and drove it partway into the garage, about to the windshield. I got out and ran around to the passenger side of the car. I walked up to the front fender of the car. There was a large grinder setting a few inches from the fender. I bent down between the grinder and the fender to pick up a block of wood on the floor. Suddenly there was a large bang of thunder and a huge crash of lighting.

My mother came from the house just screaming are you OK? She said when it thundered a large ball of fire came down on the back of the car. I stood up and told her I guess I'm OK.

We talked for a few minutes and my back and chest started to tighten up. She said we better go to the hospital.

By the time we got to the hospital, about six miles, my chest was tightening up and it was getting difficult to breath. From emergency they took me directly to radiology for x-rays, then back to emergency. I found I had to breath with my stomach my chest was getting very sore.

The doctor came in and sat down. She asked what happened, Mother explained about the ball of fire coming down on the car, I told her how I was bent down between the fender and the grinder. I told her I was wet and the car was wet also. The lightning apparently struck the car and went thru me under my left armpit and out my right armpit, and probably passed through my heart. Because I was so wet, the lightening went through me. The doctor said I was very lucky, if I had been a few inches away from the car, we would not be there talking.

For the next couple of weeks all I could do was sit in the rocking chair and take pain pills. It was very hard to breathe using my lungs and to use my stomach to breathe. Father was getting behind with the farm work. One day I told him if he would fill the Allis Chalmers tractor, the one with the cultivator on it – with gas, maybe I could sit on the cushion seat and drive and cultivate. I found sitting on the cushion was very relaxing and since the corn and beans were small and I needed to go slow, it was very relaxing indeed. I practically lived on that tractor after that. After a couple of weeks, the pain subsided and went away. I can still predict the weather as good as the weather bureau some times.

After some years passed I started having coughing spells. Our family physician sent me to a pulmonary physician. He would put me on the predizone series of pills. The cough would return again in a few months. He gave me several breathing tests. Several times my blood count would be low. A couple of times he prescribed oxygen at home for me. A couple of days later the blood count would be ok and he would cancel the machine.

After three years, the doctor sent me to the University Hospital in Ann Arbor. The doctor there did some tests and said there was nothing wrong with my lungs, that I had post nasal drip. He prescribed three medicines and sent me home. I did not have any more cough after that for years.

In June of 2002 on a Sunday evening at home, I started to get an uneasy feeling in my chest. It started to extend down my left arm. I went out and took an aspirin. The feeling continued to get worse. I went and laid down. After a little while I got up and told my wife, maybe she should take me to the hospital, and that maybe I was having a heart attack.

When we got to the hospital I was holding my chest; the emergency staff came running and had me lay down and a nurse put a nitro pill under my tongue. They admitted me to ICU for the night and in the morning a doctor confirmed that the tests showed I had a heart attack. They made arrangements to have me transported to Ingham Cardio Hospital in Lansing by ambulance. The doctor said we should have called an ambulance from home the night before I could have died on the way to the hospital. He said many people that have symptoms similar to me ignore them, go to bed, and never wake up. He said I was very lucky.

At Ingham hospital tests showed one of my arteries was completely blocked and another was 95% blocked. I had five stints put into my heart.

In the mid-1950's I formed a country music band: The Sun Valley boys. I was the leader of the band and played guitar, sang and called square dances and round dances. We had a guitar player who could do Elvis Presley songs, a drummer and fiddle player and an accordion player.

A local Ralston Purina feed dealer contacted us to put on a show like the Grand Ole Opera in Nashville, Tennessee. We rented the local Community Center.

Dealers and suppliers for the feed store came and set up booths to display their products. In the middle of the afternoon we had a local talent show with participants from the area performing their talents and music. The Sun Valley Boys played some songs for the audience. The people were invited back for an evening show and dancing. A huge crowd showed up and we played and sang for a while before we stopped and they cleared the dance floor. People lined up to get autographs and I don't know how many times I signed, but people said we were signing for over ½ hour. Finally we got back to playing and singing and I called several square dances.

One member of the band went into the service, another moved away, I got married – finally the band broke up. My wife and I played records for dances for a while.

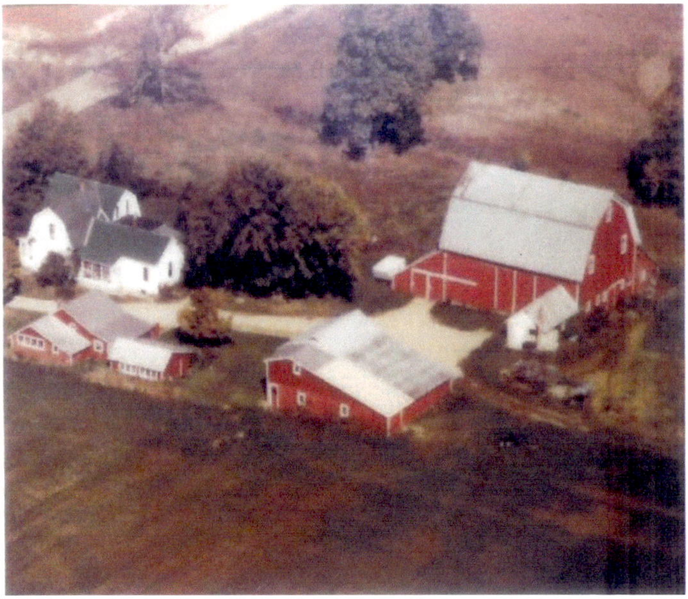

The Dumond Farm in the 1950's

CHAPTER 5

The Decision Making Years

In the fall of 1955 I went to work in a factory in Owosso for the winter. The second day a man came to me and introduced himself. He was the supervisor of the shipping department. He said he had watched me work the day before and wanted me to come and work for him in the shipping department.

My job was going throughout the factory with a cart and picking up the finished parts and taking them to the shipping department. The company made interior trim parts for the automobile industry. I would go to the end of each production lines inspector, and pick up the finished product and take it to shipping department to be put into the proper containers. I would then put together orders for shipping out to various factories.

As I went throughout the factory picking up parts, there was one red headed inspector that seemed to give me problems all the time. After several weeks I asked her if she would like to go out on a date, she said "yes". I found out later that she had a bet with just about everyone in the factory that she would get a date with me.

Eventually I proposed to her and in 1958 Mary Alice Serr and David Dudley Dumond were married. In 1960 we purchased our house in Corunna. It was a fine home built back in the 1860's.

In September of 1956, the Farm County Agent came out to the farm and brought a man with him. He introduced himself as being from the Michigan Farm Journal magazine in Lansing. They were doing a feature article on young farm boys and their future in farming. He said I was a very good example and would like to have me and my father Hugh's picture on the front cover along with an article. He took the picture and we sat for a while and discussed my options and the future.

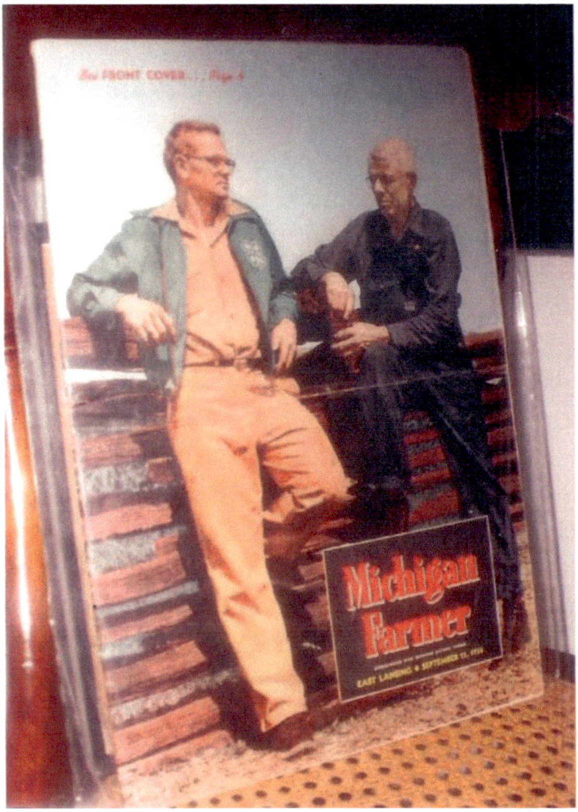

Michigan Farmer

East Lansing, MI * Sept. 15, 1956

FRONT COVER of MICHIGAN FARMER

Meet Hugh Dumond and his son David, appearing on the front cover. The Dumonds are farming in central Shiawassee County. A farm of 70 acres has been in the family for over 100 years. In additional 180 acres they rent makes a total of 250 acres devoted to general farming.

When this picture was taken the men were discussing an important question. David is 24 years old. He took vocational agriculture in high school and was active in FFA. While he didn't belong to a 4-H club he has been a volunteer leader for the past 4 years. In 1951 he attended Michigan State University for an 8-week short course in agriculture, and David and his dad have had a very satisfactory father-son partnership the past 2 years. But David is looking into the future. One of these days he expects to get married. When that time comes he realizes that their present operation just isn't big enough to support 2 families. They haven't the capital to buy more land, and he fails to see much profit in renting.

David is pondering the wisdom of his leaving the farm for a job in town. Neither of the men like the idea, but they're facing cold facts. Hugh is still young enough to handle the home farm, plus a few rented acres, keeping the present 14-cow dairy herd. Then later, when dad and mother decide to retire, David might return with his family to take over. That's what's they're talking about.

Even though I decided to leave the farm. My wife Mary and all of our children continued to go out to the farm and drive tractors and working on the farm.

My mother Marjorie passed away in 1978 and my father Hugh passed away in 1990. I took over the farm and a friend of ours, started working the land for me. Our son Todd got married and moved on the farm to raise his family. He is buying the farm on a land contract, keeping the farm in the same family. It will be in the family for 150 years in 2011.

In 1956 I took a Civil Service exam to become a State trooper. They were out of candidates for future schools. By the time I completed the class, the legislature had put on a freeze on all new hiring and were not hiring at the time. I came home and in December of 1956 I went to work on the Shiawassee County Sheriff Department as a deputy. They wanted me because of having gone to the State Police School.

I got to do everything, operate the radio, patrol out on the road, answering complaints, working accidents and doing investigations of crimes committed. I was an examiner for the State of Michigan, and wrote drivers licenses for years.

The first night on the road patrol, I went with another officer. About 9 o'clock he stopped at an all night restaurant in Owosso for supper. When we went out he tossed me the keys and said you know how to drive. I got in and started the patrol car. All of a sudden, a siren started blowing. He started to laugh.

The siren button was under my foot. I worked on every shift over the next few years. Mostly alone and sometimes with another officer. We were responsible for any and all calls while working. One Sunday while patrolling on a state expressway, a sports car went by me going very fast. I took pursuit, the car was going over 100 mph. I radioed in to the office, to call the state police, in Flint. When we got to our county line, it slowed down, and exited heading north on a state highway. I slowed down and exited behind the car. As I passed over the expressway I blew a front tire. Seconds after going so fast, over 100 miles per hour, the wrecker came and changed the tire. I had a lot of time to think about my family.

I got a letter from the State Police, they were back to hiring. They wanted me to report for a three-week brush up course. I told them that I was working for the Shiawassee County Sheriff Department and was no longer interested.

I worked many bad fatal accidents while in patrol. They did not seem to bother me, I had a job to do and didn't think about it. The only call I handled while on patrol that bothered me, was when I got a call to go to a 9-year-old boy missing at a gravel pit.

When I got there people were walking the fields and men were in the water searching for the boy. The lady that lived in front of the gravel pit, had the boy's mother up in her house. After about an hour the boy was found drowned in the gravel pit.

The County Coroner was there. He came over to me and asked if I was ready to go see his mother and finish our reports. I said let's go and get it over. When we finished with our reports I got in the patrol car and started in to the office. I radioed in and said I was on my way in. They radioed back and told me to hurry in, TV and news reporters were there waiting. When I got home after work I was sick and couldn't eat for days. The boy was the same age as one of my sons.

At the time there were no labor unions for the sheriff department's employees, they were hired at the discretion of the sheriff. When the election came around the current sheriff decided to retire. One of the deputies decided to run and a man who was a justice of peace for a number of years decided to run for sheriff also. Each officer was contacted by the candidates and asked if you were for or against him? Are you going to support me or not? Eight of the deputies were for the officer and eight were for the justice of peace. Fortunately, I had supported the man that won the election for sheriff.

The new sheriff came to my house one evening. He asked if I would be willing to take over the department at midnight New Years Eve. I told him I would be honored to do it. He said he was promoting me to Sergeant as I was the best qualified officer he had, and he knew the department would be in good hands for the night.

At midnight on New Years I went down to the jail and parked in back. In a few minutes the Sheriff arrived with his family and some friends. At 12:00 midnight the clock on the courthouse started to strike. We got out of our cars and went inside the jail. The Deputy behind the desk got up and went to congratulate the sheriff. I went around and sat down at the radio. About that time the old sheriff and his wife came out of their quarters in the building. He walked up to the new sheriff and shook his hand. He said "I suppose this is the time for turning over the keys." The new sheriff said "you can give them to this officer he will be running the department for me, the rest of the night." I was on cloud nine.

One night while on patrol another officer and I stopped for supper at a restaurant over on the west side of our county. When our supper came the phone rang, they had a call of a prowler out on the north side of our county. About 18 miles from us. I don't know to this day why, but I had a feeling we should hurry. I drove with lights and siren on. When we got to the address, there was a car that had hit their driveway and rolled over, ending up in the ditch in front of their house. The people who lived in the house were old and did not know what the noise was. The driver of the car was a young boy who lived around the corner. He was completely under the car. We called for a wrecker and ambulance. When they arrived and moved the car so we could get to him he was dead. The people were devastated. We had to go around the corner and notify his parents.

Five years later I left the sheriff's department as a Sergeant. The pay was not great and having seven mouths to feed at home times were tough. I had spent 10 years as a Deputy Sheriff. During that time I handled fatal accidents, murders, suicides, and just about everything in between. However, I enjoyed it very much.

Mary continued to work in the factory until our first son (Timothy) was born. Next came no. 2 son (Thomas) and no. 3 son (Todd). Finally twins; a girl (Tamara) and her twin brother (Terry). Bingo we figured out what caused it all. My mother has a twin sister, and my father had twin brothers that were still born at birth. Five children in four years, makes for a very close family. They are all now living within 1½ hour from us.

I have always said Mother makes the rules and I enforce them.

As our sons and daughter grew up, I got involved in scouting. I took over as cub master of our pack 77 cub scouts. In 1969 our city of Corunna was celebrating its 100th year as a city. I took the full week off as vacation, to celebrate in the festival. I grew an Abe Lincoln beard for the festival. Mary made clothing for the kids and a dress for herself. I wore a derby and long black coat like Abe Lincoln. All week long we walked around town. Everyone was having a great time celebrating,

By that time we had over 120 boys in the Cub Scout pack. They were very active in 9 cub dens and 2 webelos dens. One day the city had a huge parade. Our Cub Scout pack took up an entire block in the parade. Mary worked on several committees.

On the final day they judged various contests. Our family won a plaque for the best dressed family of the week. There were 32 entries for the Abe Lincoln beard contest, I won the plaque for first place.

As time came and went, the boys got involved in boy scouting, including weekend camp outs. My wife Mary and daughter Tamara were left home on weekends. We decided to buy two canoes and a camper, and the whole family could go together. As the boys got older and were in many more activities we gave up scouting.

We vacationed in Northern Michigan almost every summer, when time allowed. We loved to go canoeing on the river in Traverse City. Mary's aunt lived on East Bay, and we would campout in her back yard, going swimming in the bay and fishing.

One summer we went on a trip to Boston, Washington DC and Gettysburg for a week with the camper. We had a very nice trip. It was very hot that summer.

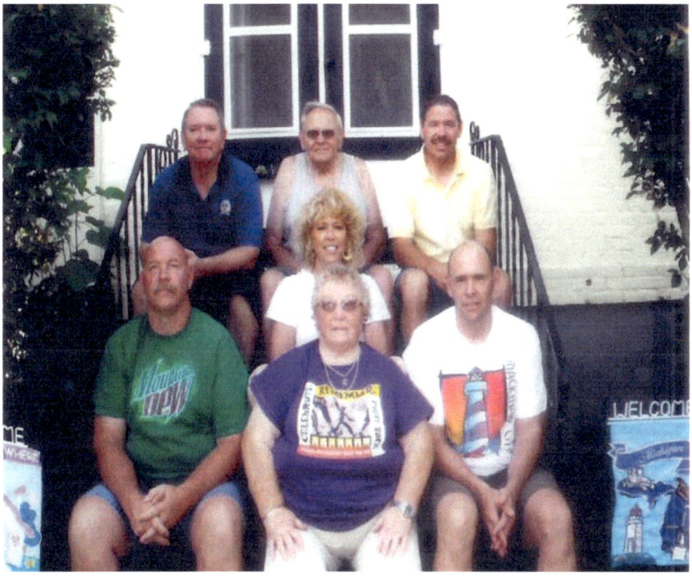

Timothy David Terry

Tamara

Todd Mary Thomas

After the kids left home to go to College and to get married, we decided to get tickets for Michigan State University football and hockey games. We would tailgate with several family members and friends, before the games. Mary and I went with friends to national final hockey games, in Cincinnati, Ohio; Milwaukee, Wisconsin; Boston Massachusetts; Providence, Rhode Island; and Buffalo, New York. Because the games were in the month of April, and usually nothing was open yet for the summer. We would end up going to the zoo in each city for a day.

My wife Mary had a breast removed in 1987, from cancer. She is doing fine since the surgery.

I went to the hospital for a stress test in 1997 for my heart. The test went well. They took me in for an x-ray of my heart. When the test was finished I lay down for a few minutes. Finally the nurse said I could leave. I felt okay and walked down the hall to the elevator. I punched the button, went into the elevator and punched the 1st floor button the door closed. When the door opened on the first floor for a woman, I lay on the floor passed out. When I came to, the elevator was full of doctors, orderlies and nurses. They took me to emergency. I was okay by then and they sent me home.

I served as a councilperson for our City of Corunna for four years. I was on the planning commission before that. I am on the Economic Development Commission and the Zoning Board of Appeals now.

We have twelve grandchildren that participate in sports; football, baseball, soccer, track and field, basketball, and tennis. Two of the boys have black belts in Tekondo, and some are wrestlers. When someone calls and says they are going to do something, do we want to go? We say our bags are always packed.

In high school I had taken bookkeeping and typing. I looked for a job in an office. I got hired as a cost accountant at a local factory. After working there for a short time the accounting supervisor asked me to come into his office. He said he liked my work and wondered if I was interested in getting more education? I told him I was but couldn't afford it. He said he had a friend who had taken courses with a correspondence school in Scranton Pennsylvania, and got a good education. If I was interested the company was willing to pay for the tuition. He would be my tutor and help me if I had any problems. I enrolled in the International Correspondence School in Scranton, Pennsylvania. Every evening it was out to the kitchen table and weekends at the kitchen table studying for me.

Mary would work with the five children, as I studied in the kitchen. Two years later I had an Associates Degree in Financial Management. My boss said he had a college degree, and I had things he did not get in college. He felt I had gotten an excellent education in finance and business management. I was an accountant at the factory for 7 years.

I went to work for Lansing General Hospital. I was the accounting supervisor. I was in charge of the business office, accounts payable, payroll, accounts receivable, collections, and financial statements.

I left there after 7 years. The price of gasoline went way over $1.00 per gallon and I was driving over 90 miles per day to work. A local factory near home needed an accounting manager. They matched the benefits and pay from the hospital, so I left the hospital and drove only 10 miles each day to work. After about 5 years things started to slow down at the factory and I got laid off.

I drew unemployment for a while, and finally got a job working for a handicapped facility that worked with handicapped people. Training them in new skills and working with their hands.

My job was finding work that these people could do with their hands. Two days a week I would travel, calling on factories and businesses, looking for work for the handicapped workers. The other days I stayed in the facility working with the people.

As time went along and calling on these businesses, I ran into lots of companies that would say we wish there was a place where we could send work like inspection, assembly, and packaging out to be done. Then they could put their people to work making more products.

With all of my experience in factory accounting and business, I started thinking about a business that would do these tasks for the industries.

CHAPTER 6

Our Family Business

With pen in hand I started to put together a plan to start our own business. In 1988 I registered Skilled Services Incorporated with the State of Michigan. My wife and all five of our sons and daughter were officers of the corporation.

I put together a working five year plan that projected what should be an estimated balance sheet and profit and loss, for the corporation the first five years of operation. I found a factory in the Corunna City Industrial Park that was empty. A corporation still had 1½ years on their lease, so we subleased the buildings for the last 18 months. I applied for a government small business loan for $100,000 for five years. The bank said it would take four to six weeks to come through.

We were starting to locate some work for us to do. I went to the City of Corunna economic development committee and borrowed $25,000 dollars for 5 years at a very low interest rate so we could start operations.

We started packaging sanding papers, grinding wheels and Knife sharpening blocks, for a local factory, that manufactured them.

We had no employees so our family members and friends came down evenings and weekends to help us get started. Gradually we brought in more work, and started hiring new employees.

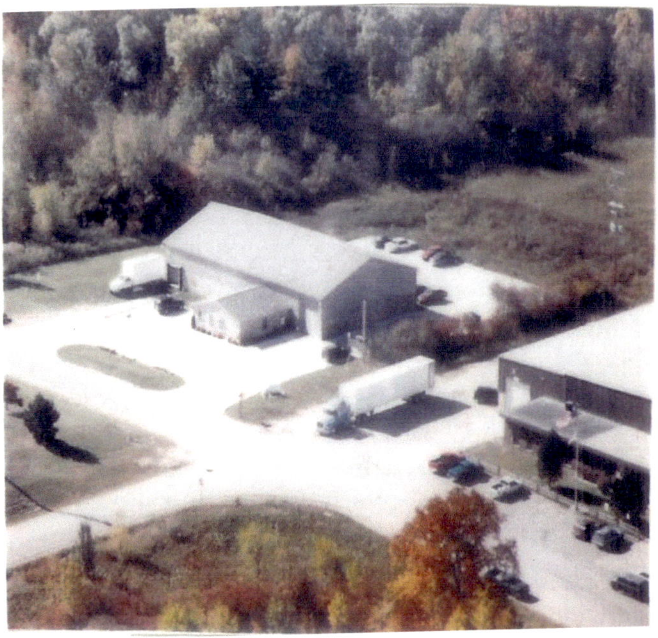

Skilled Services, Inc. Owosso, MI

Founded in 1986

Our son Terry was a licensed building contractor, and built us several work tables 4ft. by 8ft. and 4ft. high. He also built benches for the employees and we were off and going. We found that the retired people were very pleased to be doing something. They would come in early and make the coffee and sit around talking before starting work.

A company that cut glass, for other industries contacted us and said they cut wooden blocks for putting in boxes, to put sheets of glass in to keep them from breaking during shipping. They would like to get this job out of their factory. I purchased an industrial table saw, for the job. We would pick up bunks of the lumber from them and pallets of boxes to put the cut blocks in. We delivered the finished products to them and picked up more material for our plant.

I purchased a used truck, and had a new 50ft.box built for it. It was loading dock high. We also bought two forklifts. One was used and one was new. I purchased a new pickup with a topper for my personal use and for the plants use also.

We did some work for a factory about 20 miles away. Mary would use the pickup and deliver product to them two or three times a week.

Another company manufactured small metal blocks that went into seat belts for the automobile industry. They were the thing that locked your seat belt during an accident. Being a safety item they had to be looked at one at a time. We inspected thousands of them every day. They would deliver several barrels of them to us every day and picked up the inspected barrels.

Our shifts were set up, 7 a.m. to 11 a.m. and 11 a.m. to 3 p. m. When we got very busy we worked from 3 p.m. to 7 p.m. also.

The people had social security insurance and just needed more money to pay bills. We found housewives would also come to work. They would get their kids to school and come to work for four hours. They would pick the kids up on their way home.

These people were excellent workers, they had put in their time, were in good health and just needed something to do. We had employees working for us for 12 and 14 of our 18 years in business.

Sometimes we would get in a new job from a factory to do, and one of our employees would say that they used to do that job when they worked for that company. We would say that's good you can show us how to do it.

An excellent job came to us from a factory just down the street from us. They were making laser machines for industries. Every time they shipped a machine out they included a set-up kit along with the machine. They gave me a list of their suppliers, and what parts I needed to put into the setup kits.

I purchased all of the parts that were needed to put into a setup kit for them. We built a tool crib in one corner of the factory, installed shelving and made this the place to assemble the set-up kits. We could shut the door and keep other personal out.

In 1996 we bought property over in an Owosso Industrial Park and built a new 100 ft. by 300 ft, factory with a 50 ft. by 50 ft office on the front. Our son Terry designed the building. The building was contracted out, and Terry built the office and the rest of our family helped one way or another. We had came full circle and ended up in our factory.

A factory we did work for occasionally, when they had a job we could do, sent their factory manager over one day. They were getting ready to install new machinery for the next year's auto industry, and wondered if we could take the old machines and finish out the model year. He said they would set up the machines in our factory and would come and train our employees. If we had a breakdown or whatever, their maintenance people would come and keep us going.

Some of the machines needed a good air supply to operate. I found a large compressor used and bought it. In order to produce their volume of work we had to put on a third shift, 3 p.m. to 7 p.m. Our son Todd came to supervise the third shift for about two months. We hired more people to work that shift. There were about 15 machines.

Another job was for an outdoor furniture factory. We put together sample sales material blotches for their sales department.

In 1992 we were starting to get known in the business world. One day a man walked in and said he owned a Public Television Station in Midland Michigan. Showing at 7 a.m. on Tuesdays and again at 7 p.m. on Thursdays, he had a program called Money Matters at the station. He had heard about our factory, and would like to do a feature program about the older workers and people who worked for us, and what we were doing to help the older people. I told him I would be delighted with the idea.

He spent the day photographing the people at work. We set up a date and time for me to come up to the station in Midland. When I got there he and I sat down in a couple of lounge chairs with a lamp between us on a small table. He and I talked about how I came up with the idea of the hiring older people part time. As we talked they were showing people working in the plant. It lasted thirty minutes. He gave me a taping of the program. It is interesting to sit down and watch the program. Our son Thomas has put the program on a disk. My family will be able to show my great-grandchildren their grandpa on TV.

In 2002 I bought a new truck and had the box from the old truck put on it.

I had hired our daughter Tamara as Personnel Director and eventually promoted her to Plant Manager. She worked very well with the employees and ran a tough ship. We had two supervisors sometimes. If I walked out in the plant they would say you get back in the office and stay there.

I paid off our loans in less than four years.

One Christmas we rented a hall and put on a fine dinner for the employees, and their families. Our whole family was there to serve and wait on the employees.

Eighteen good years. The economy started to decline, some factories started closing, some were moving away. One closed its plant in the US and went back to Switzerland.

In 2005 Skilled Services Inc. paid for the Board of Directors, and their families to go to Disney World in Florida. All 24 family members were able to attend for one full week.

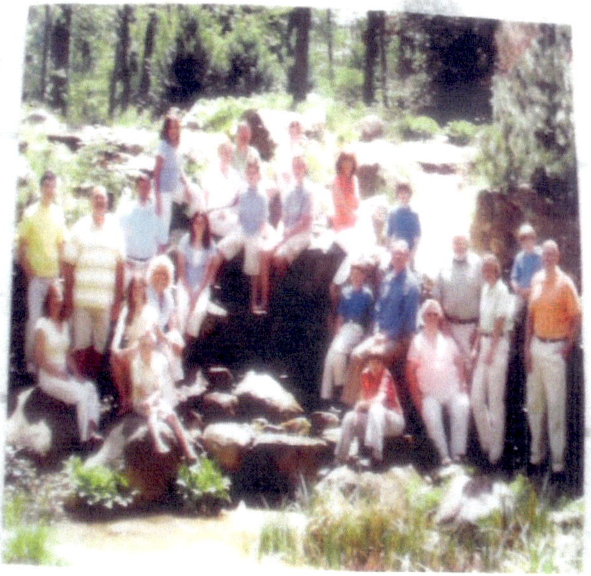

24 DUMOND FAMILY MEMBERS

(dad, mom, 4 sons, 1 daughter, 4 daughter-in-laws, 1 son-in-law, 12 grandkids)

In 2006 after eighteen good years in business, work was falling off. Some factories we were doing work for were closing.

We had a Board of Directors meeting. They said you have had an excellent run and maybe we should sell everything, including the building and retire. In 2006 we sold the building and all of the equipment.

June 2006, I went into the hospital and had a St. Jude Pacemaker defibrillator installed. Six months later in 2007, I went into the Owosso Memorial Hospital. They hooked me up to a machine, stopped my heart, and the pacemaker kicked in and started my heart. The pacemaker was working fine.

CHAPTER 7

Those Retirement Years

September 2008 I went to Ingham Medical Osteopathic Hospital to have a total right shoulder replaced. The Osteopathic Doctor called it a reverse procedure, developed over in France about 5 years earlier, they replace the total ball and socket. It is a new procedure here in the States. During surgery, my heart started to fail. A cardio physician was called over from the Cardiology unit of the hospital. My shoulder surgery was completed. They called for an ambulance to come and take me over to the cardio hospital. A nurse came and told my wife where to go at the heart unit.

I was put on a machine for my heart, and in a medical induced coma, until they could find out what was happening with my heart. I was kept in this coma for over 2 1/2 weeks. My wife and family members traveled 2 hours every day to see me. The doctor that did my shoulder said he came over every day and she was there always. Mary told me probably many different times 5 or 6 doctors came in and looked at my chart and checked my condition. A nurse came in and told Mary that Medicare was going to stop my hospital charges. They were making out paperwork to send me to an extended care facility, near our home. Mary said the 6 doctors came in to check on me. They started talking together and were getting somewhat concerned. Mary said the head surgeon came over to her and said we are going into surgery immediately, my heart was failing and we are going to lose him. She started calling my family and telling them, so they could come. A nurse came and took Mary to the surgery waiting room and stayed until some of our family got there. My blood oxygen had dropped to less than 50 when they took the oxygen away from me.

The surgeon came in after the surgery and said they found a hole between the right ventricular and the left ventricular in my heart, and it was allowing the good blood and the bad blood to flow back and forth. It appeared to have enlarged some and was causing my trouble.

I told him about being struck by lightning 55 years ago, and the lightning passing thru my heart. Probably that had something to do with the oxygen problems I had over the years.

He said he had opened up my heart and fixed the hole up, I should have no more problems.

Three days after surgery the Doctor came in my room, and asked how I was feeling. I stood up and thanked him for saving my life. I told him I had been up walking. He said insurance was going to stop and if I felt good enough he would sign my release papers. He said for me to contact his office for an appointment in 2 weeks.

I called Mary to come and get me. Riding home everything seemed strange to me. When I got home she turned into the driveway, I looked at her and said why are we stopping here. She said this is where we live this is our house. Nothing seemed right, it was not my house, everything was strange to me. I had lost many years off my life. It took about three days before everything came back to me.

I started on home care therapy, a nurse came every other day to check me out, plus a therapist came to get me started on physical therapy. The osteopathic doctor prescribed a month of outpatient therapy in Owosso.

After 1 week and 3 treatments I still could not raise my arm above my head. We went back to the Doctor. They took several x-rays again, the doctor came in and sat down and massaged his chin. He said the ball in my shoulder, had came out of the socked. Mary said while I lay in the hospital in the coma two orderlies would come in regularly and move me around. They were treating both of my arms the same to move me and lift me up. The doctor said he would need to take me back into surgery. If he could manipulate the ball back in place with the x-ray that would be fine. If not he would need to go back in and put it in place. He got the ball back in without surgery.

We are kept busy keeping up our home both inside and outside. We take pride in how nice our lawn looks. We get involved with grandsons and granddaughters with sports like, soccer, football, baseball, wrestling, track and field, tennis and basketball, also band, chorus and special events. We are very proud of all of our family no matter what they are involved with.

We follow Michigan State University and Corunna sporting events.

We decorate inside and outside every holiday, especially Christmas where we have many blowups and lights all around our property. We have many cars driving around every night looking at our decorations. People we see out in public tell us how nice our house looks all decorated up.

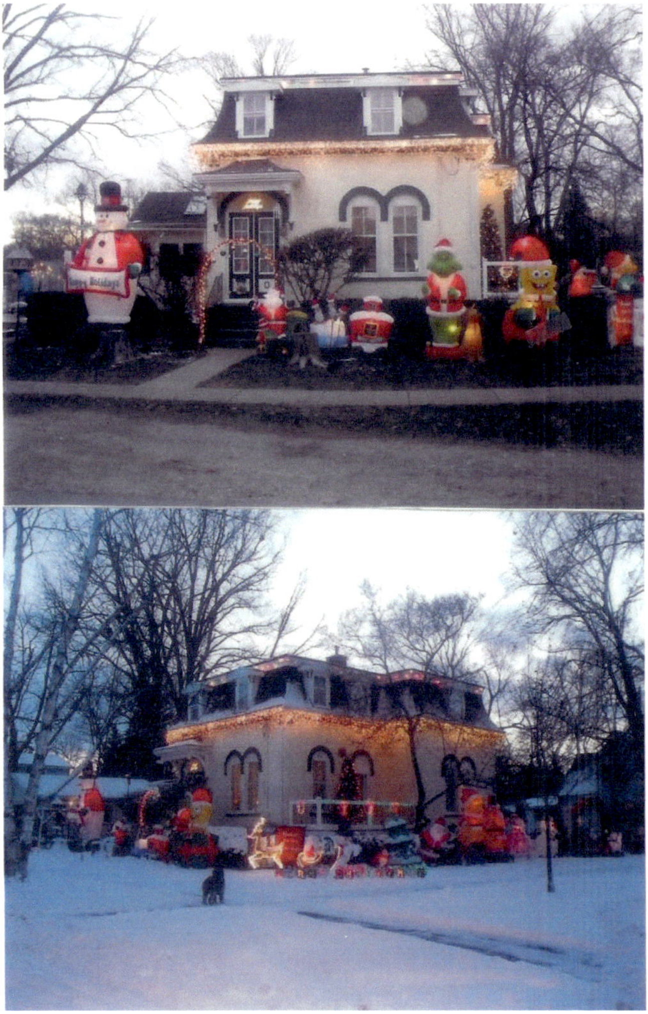

Our House Christmas 2010

We have a fireplace insert for burning wood in the winter. We cut wood during the spring and summer to burn in the winter.

I have always had a dog. Several years ago after our two Pekinese dogs died, Mary said I could not have another dog, we were gone too much. Seven years ago on fathers' day the whole family came home. We were all sitting out in the yard. Tamara and Terry left in the car and were gone for a long time. I didn't know where they went. Someone said they went out to Meijers. Finally they came back. Tamara got out and came over to me with a small puppy. I looked at Mary and she said isn't he cute. I knew right then I could keep him. He was a pure bred English Cocker Spaniel. Every one tried to think of a name for him. The kids said when they were in school everyone would say "here comes the Duwees". So we decided to name him Duwee Lapew Dumond.

I started to train him. He knows the boundary lines of our property, a fence, an alley, and two streets. We live on a corner and have a large yard. His job is keeping all animals and birds out of our yard. He will chase them to the edge of the streets and stop. He knows not to go out in the street.
He will watch for the paperboy to come and bring the paper into the house. If he goes outside and in the afternoon, he will go up on the front porch to see if the paper is there. He will go to the back door, if we do not see him, he will take it and lay it in the yard. When we go to the door and say has the paper come yet? He will go out where he put it and bring it in. He gets three dog cookies for bringing in the paper. If you go into the living room he will be laying down with one foot on top and one foot under the paper. Enough as to say where is my treat. He knows my complete routine and what I am going to do next.

When I get up in the morning, he goes into the bathroom, waiting for me to come in. When Mary gets a meal ready, she will tell him to come in and get me. If I do not see him he will bark. We can let him out and know he will stay in our yard. He will smell around to see if anything has been in our yard.

He has grown up with 12 grand children and loves kids. He will bark when someone walks by. If he does not know them he will shy away until he gets to know them. When squirrels come in the yard he will bark at them. He will sit by the tree or pole, until they leave our property. This past summer he caught 6 young opossums. I always go outside with him at night. He keeps an eye on me and where I am. I do not want him to get into trouble with another dog or some animal. He sleeps beside our bed. If I get up during the night he goes to see where I'm going, he usually knows. Where ever I go my buddy goes with me even in the car or truck.

He loves honey roasted peanuts. Every afternoon around suppertime he will come to me begging, it's time for peanuts. We will have some peanuts, and play ball with him and then he will go outside. That's his routine just like clockwork. If he wants something, like go outside, and we ignore him, he will go and sit right in front of the TV, to get our attention. Maybe it's time for peanuts or for whatever.

When I get his leash, he gets excited, he knows we are going for a walk. When we come to a street to cross he will stop until I say ok for him to cross. Mary is gone a lot so Duwee and I are buddies.

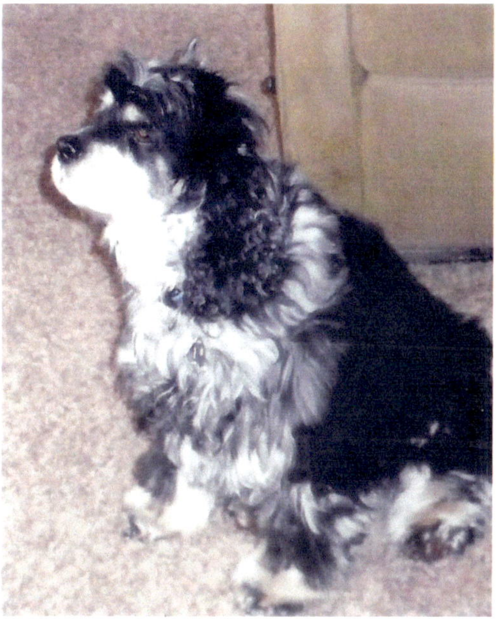

Duwee Lapew Dumond

Made in the USA
Monee, IL
09 November 2026

67377597R00036